The Illustrated Guide to Mastering Bine Broth for a Healthier
You
Or
How To Make Bone Broth that Gels

By

Matthew Frederickson

Congratulations. If you are looking for a guide to making bone broth, broth that turns to gel, and provides the healthy nutrients you need, then you have come to the right place. In this guide, I will walk you through the process of making good bone broth, step-by-step, so that you get gel – every time.

I am assuming you already know why it's good for you – you just need to know how to make it. That's exactly what this guide will provide for you. I appreciate you purchasing this book, and I believe, that if you follow my directions, you'll quickly become a bone broth making master. Enough with this – let's get started.

What You Need

There are a few thing you need to make bone broth. You need either:

- An 8-quart Instapot

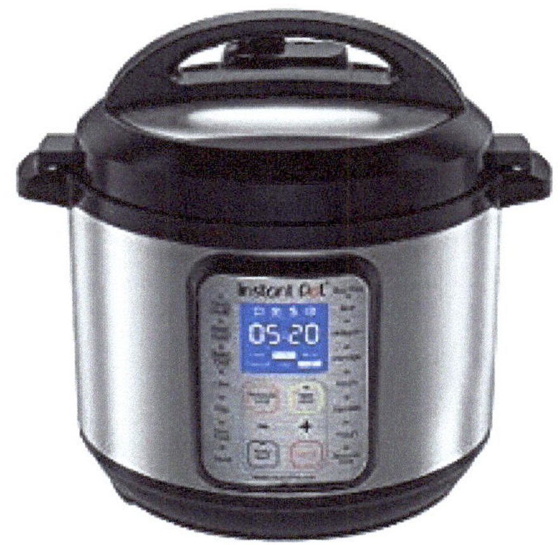

- And/or an 8-quart slow cooker

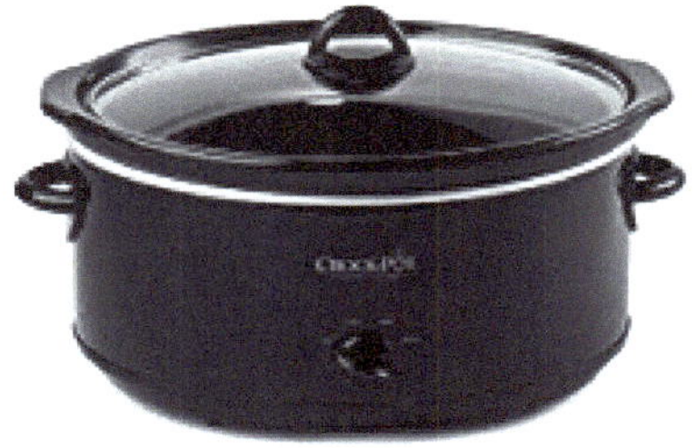

- And/or a 12-quart stock pot

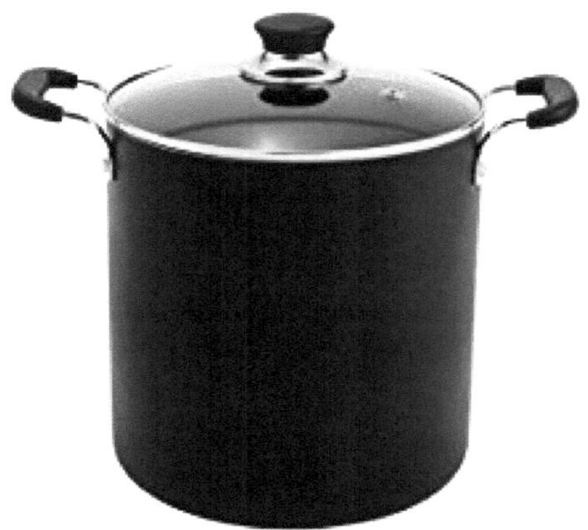

You will also need:

- A strainer (we like the one with the lip so it sets nicely on the large bowl we strain the broth into)

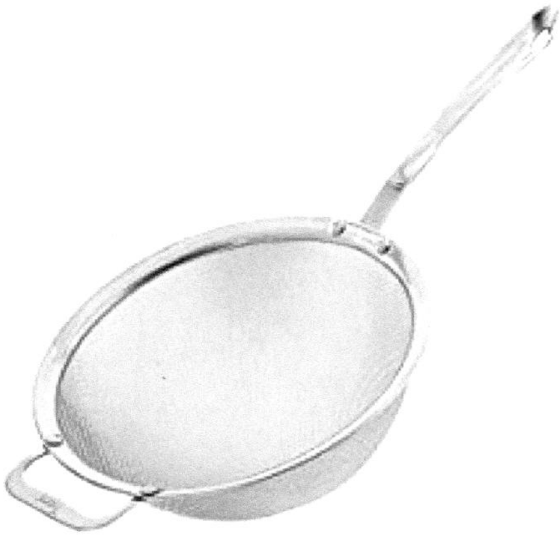

- A ladle

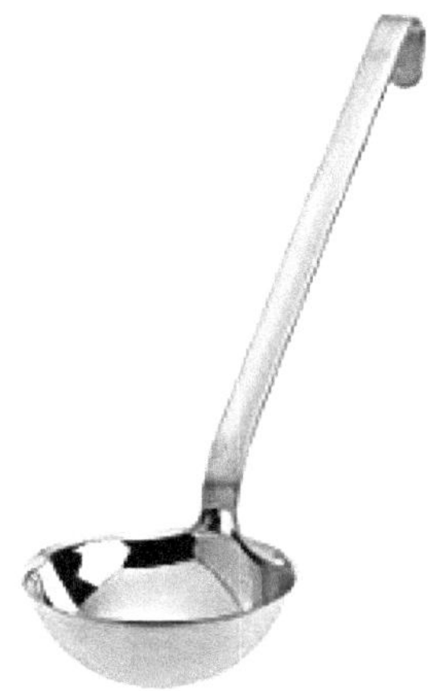

- Several bowls of various sizes

    o   A big bowl to strain the broth into from your cooking pot

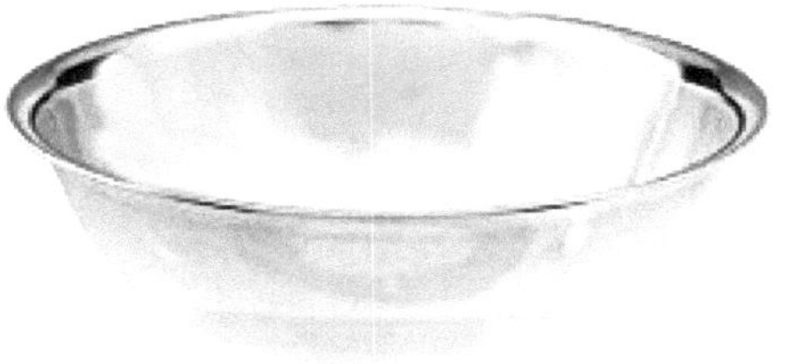

    o   Small bowls to aid the cooling process

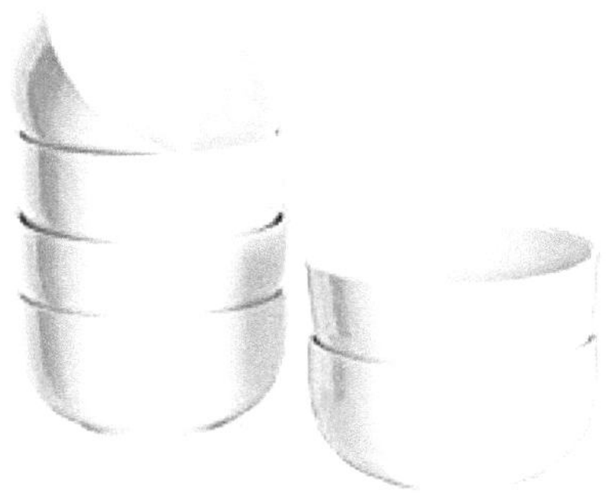

- Glass jars to store the broth (we use quart size canning jars)

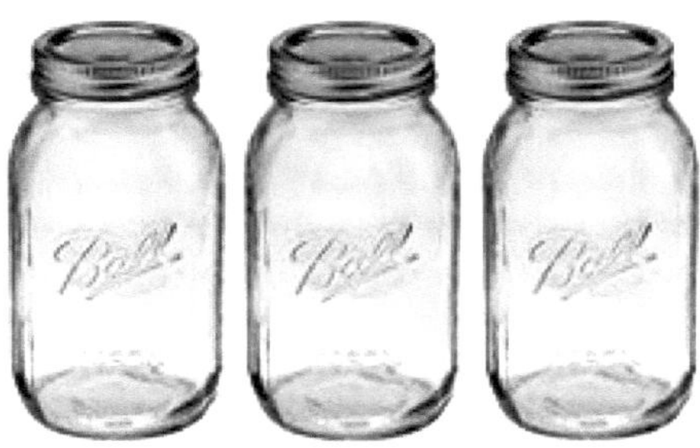

Nice to haves:

- Apron – the broth will stain your clothes, so an apron is suggested

- Trivets or cork boards to set all the bowls and pots on

- Sticky notes to place on the lids to indicate the date you bottled the broth (we reuse the jars and lids)

We use BOTH an Instapot and a crockpot. I'll explain why when I get into the actual process, but it allows us to move from the first batch to making the second batch.

<u>**The Ingredients**</u>

In order to make good bone broth, you need good bones. In fact, your broth will NOT gel properly if you do not have good bones. That's the secret to making good bone broth.

For beef bones, you need good, healthy bones from good, healthy cows. You need leg bones, knuckle bones, joint bones. You need a little meat on the bones. The picture below shows the different types of bones.

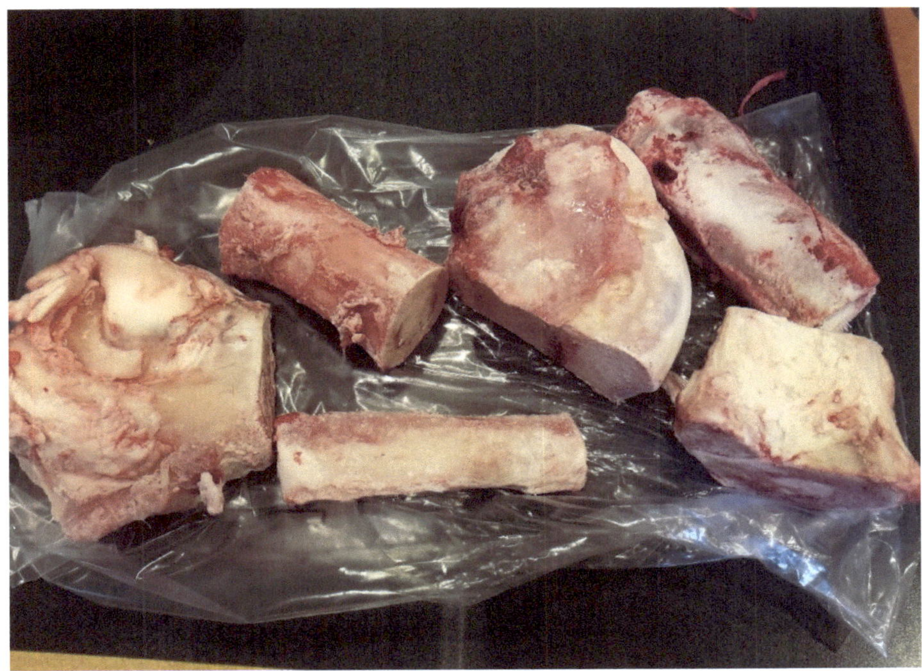

Various bone type

This is a picture of a piece of a leg bone. Notice the marrow inside the bone on the right-hand side).

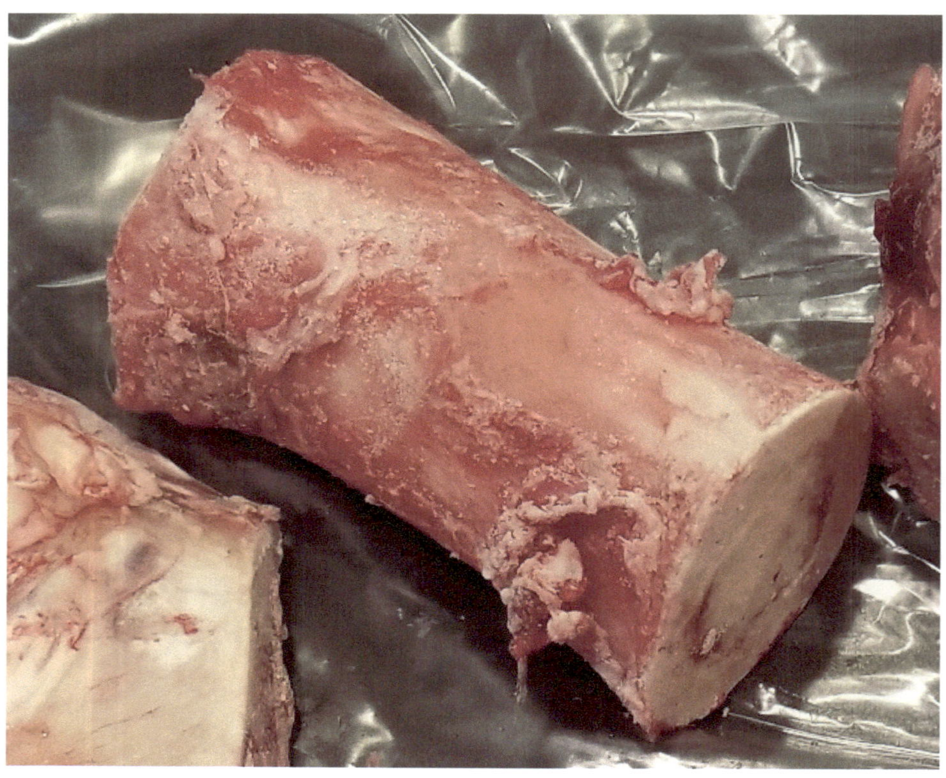

Leg bone

This is a picture of rib bones. They are stacked, so it looks like there is only one (but there are two).

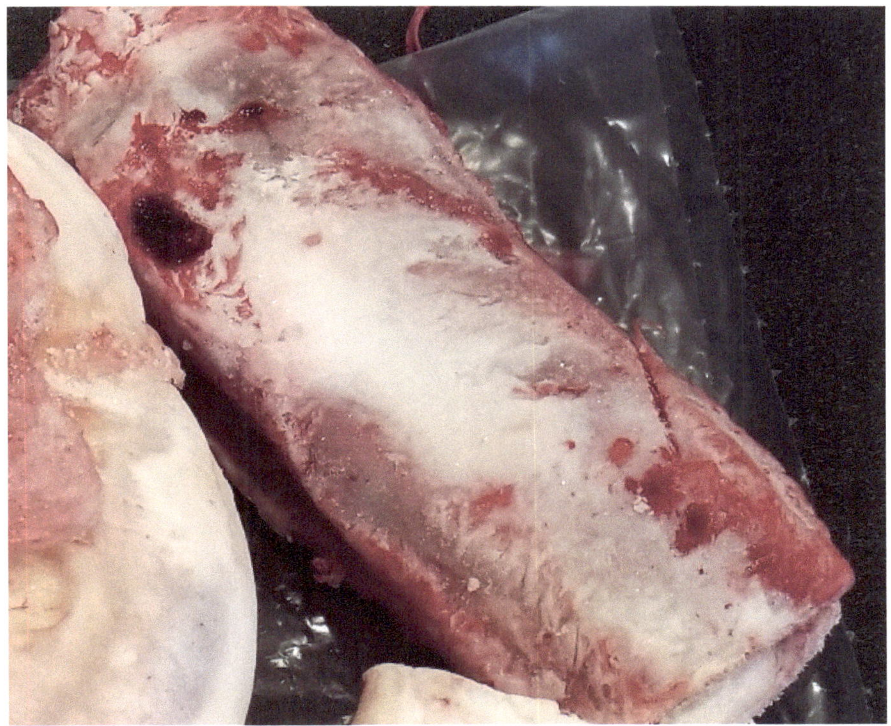

Rib bones

This is part of a joint bone.

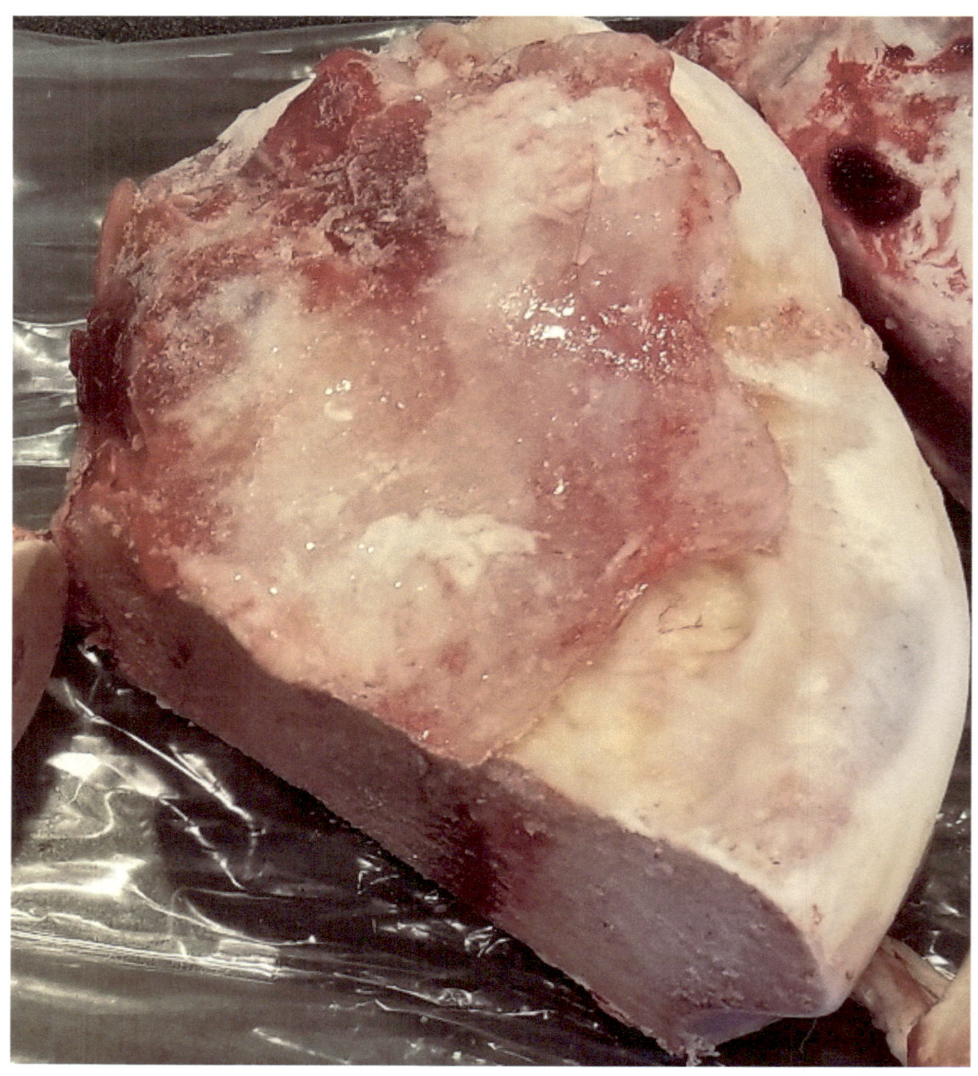

Joint bone

This is a knuckle bone:

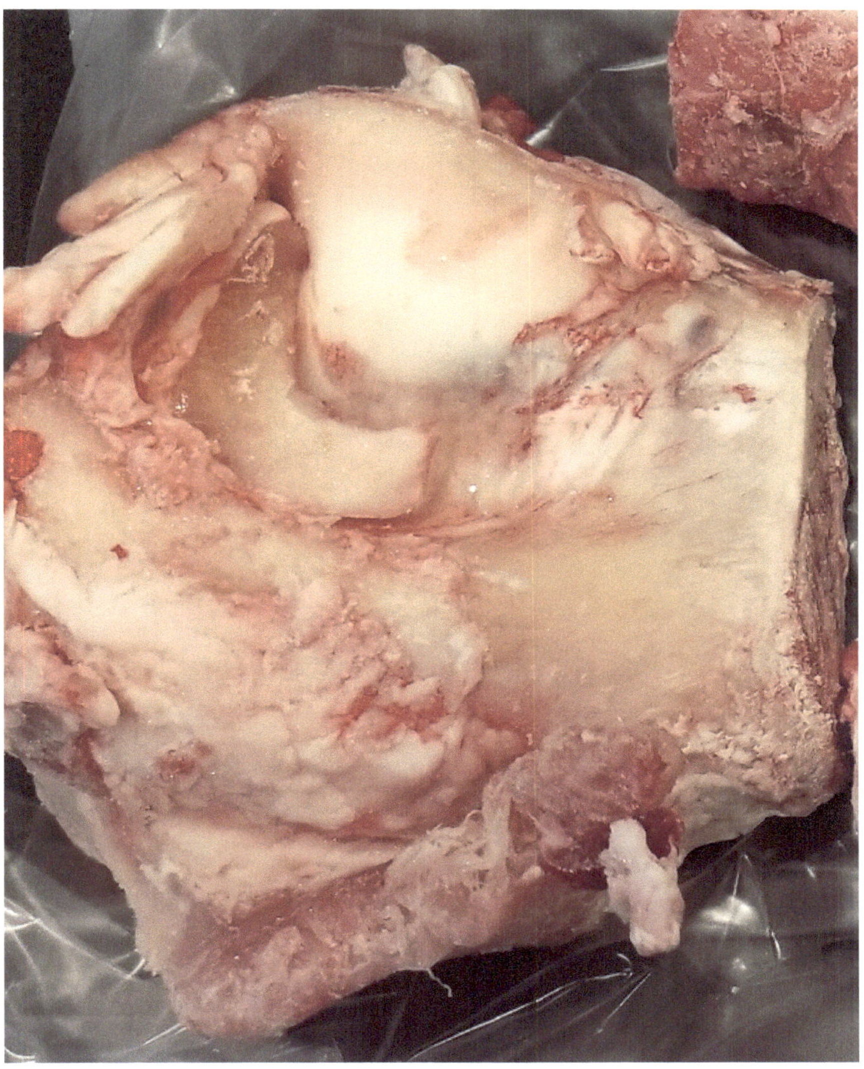

Knuckle bone

Notice that on all the bones you can still see meat and fat. The meat and fat are critical to making good bone broth.

While you can buy frozen bones in the supermarket, the best place to get bones is from a butcher shop. Most butcher shops will sell bones by the bag or box (yes, they literally give you a box of bones). When you call to order them, be explicit in what you need – a mixture of joint, knuckle and leg bones.

This applies to pork bones as well.

The easiest way to get chicken bones is to simply save the bones from when you cook whole chickens.

<u>**Ingredients for Broth**</u>

- Bones

    - 6 to 8 beef/pork bones

    OR

    - 3 to 4 sets of bones (and some skin) from whole chickens

- 2 carrots washed and chopped into 1 to 2 inch pieces or ½ bag of baby carrots (try to use whole carrots). The healthier (as in organic) the carrots, the better for you. If using whole carrots, you can peel them, or wash them well. Not peeling them provides additional nutrients.

- 2 stalks of celery, washed and cut into small 1 to 2 inch pieces.

- 1 onion, top layer peeled and cut into small chunks (I just cut mine into quarters)

- 2 or 3 cloves of garlic

- 2 tablespoons of peppercorns

- 3 to 4 bay leaves

- 2 or 3 tablespoons of apple cider vinegar (optional)

- Filtered water

How to Make Broth

This recipe is basically the same for any of the pots – Instapot, slow cooker, or stock pot. If you've tried something similar, and are not getting gel, and you are still using the same type of bones, then **add more bones** – this is what will make it gel.

1. Place 6 to 8 bones (beef or pork) in the pot. If using chicken bones, place the bones from 3 to 4 whole chickens. If using chicken bones, you may want to add chicken feet (yes, it's a thing – you can buy these at most oriental markets).

2. Wash and cut 2 stalks of celery. Add the pieces to the pot.

3. Wash and cut 2 carrots (or use ½ bag of baby carrots)   . Add them to the pot.

4. Clean and cut into quarters one medium sized yellow onion. Add that to the pot.

5. Add 3 cloves of garlic to the pot.

6. Add 2 tablespoons of peppercorns to the pot.

7. Add 3 or 4 bay leaves to the pot.

It should look something like this:

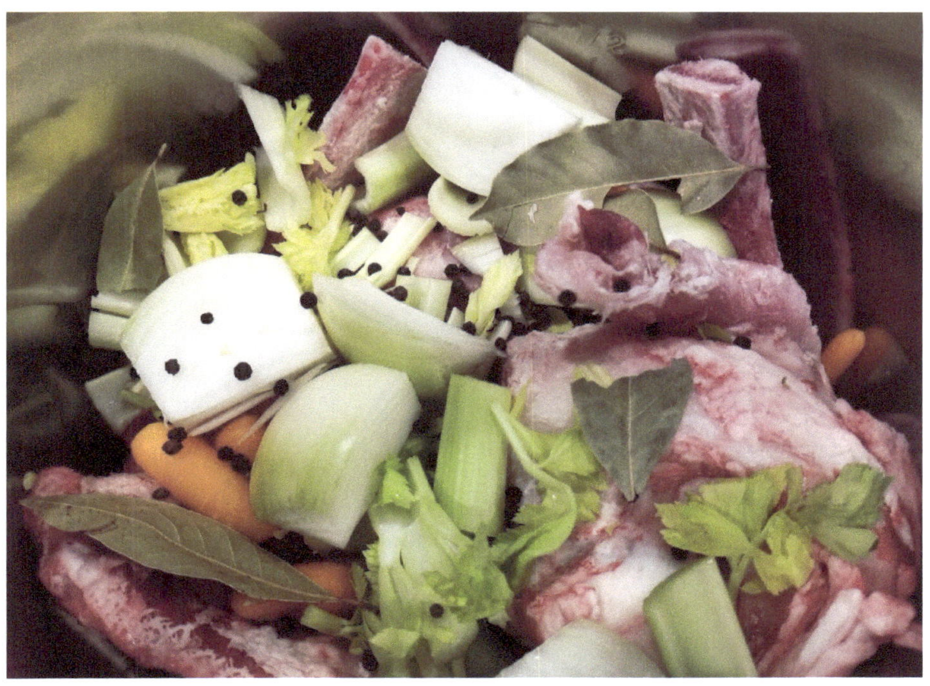

8.   Add filtered water.

        Instapot – up to the fill line

        Slow cooker or stock pot – just over the bones.

It will look like this:

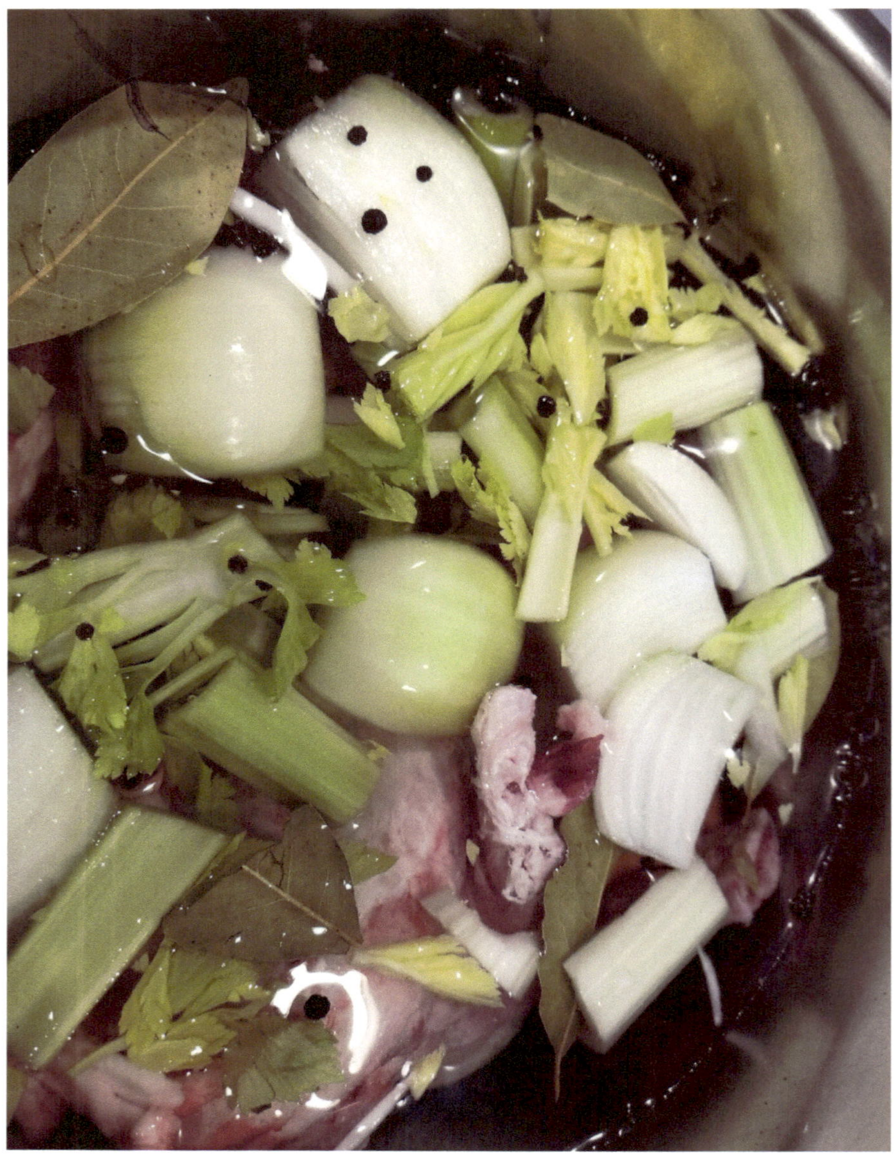

If you are having trouble getting gel, add 2 or 3 tablespoons of apple cider vinegar. This will help leach the proper minerals out of the bones. I have, when using poor bones, used as many as 5 tablespoons.

9.   Cook the broth.

        Instapot – use the Soup/Broth setting, and set the timer for 240
        minutes. When it finishes, allow it to keep cooking (after the timer
        goes off, it goes into warm mode – just leave it sit) for an additional
        4 hours. Total time: 8 hours.

        Slow Cooker – set the temperature to low, and let it cook for 48
        hours.

        Stock pot – set the temperature to low, and let it cook for 48 hours.

When it's done cooking, it will look something like this:

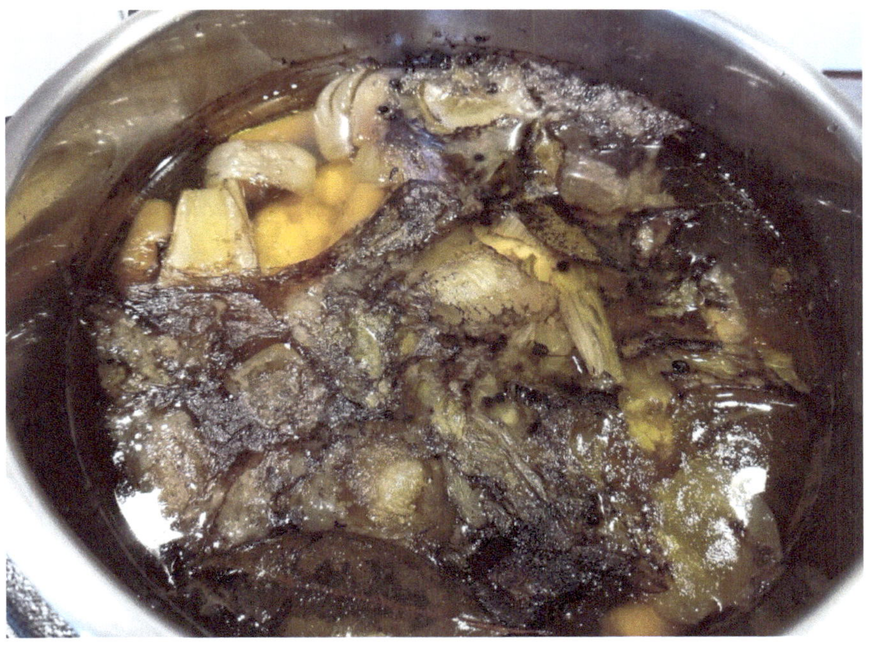

10.   Prep your area. This includes setting up a bowl to contain the broth, somewhere to put the bones, and somewhere to discard the vegetables. What we do is take the bones from the Instapot (batch 1) and place them into our slow cooker. The slow cooker becomes batch 2. We never use our bones for more than two batches.

This is what we use to hold the broth as we strain it:

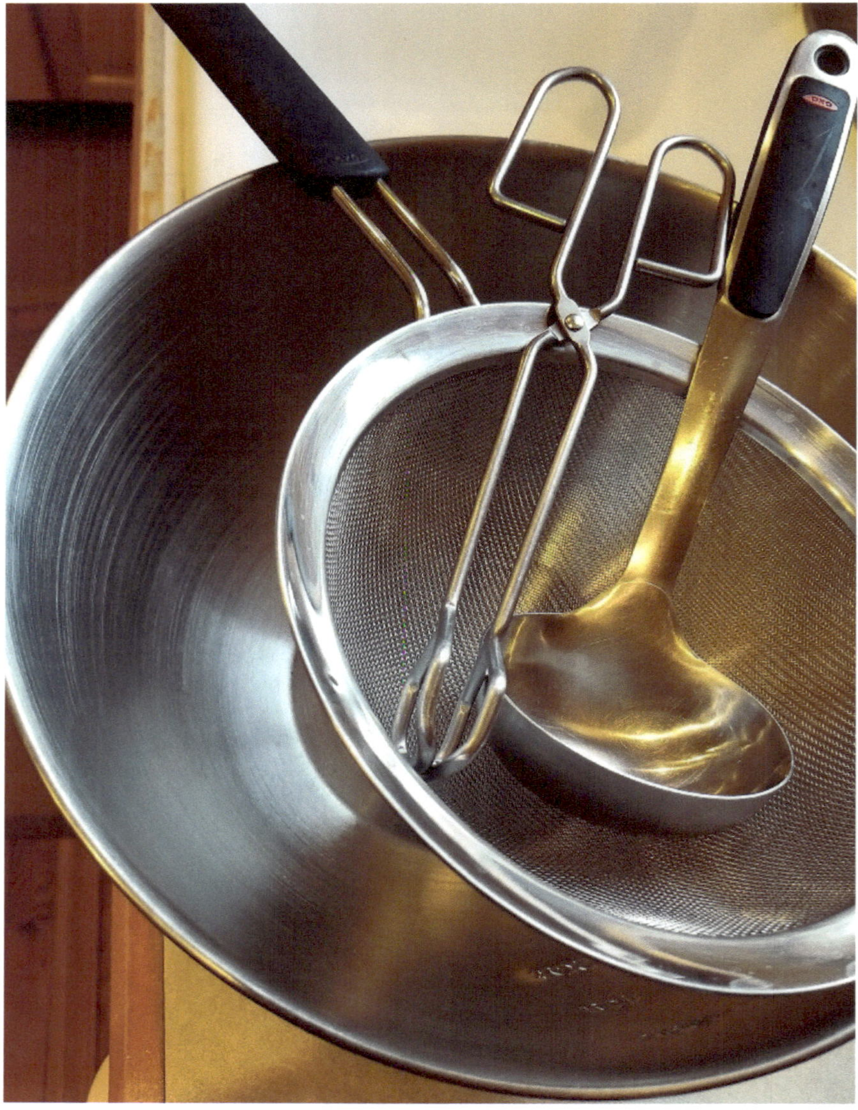

The tongs are for pulling the bones out. We always do this first, before we start straining the broth.

We also setup bowls to ladle the broth into to hasten the cooling to room temperature:

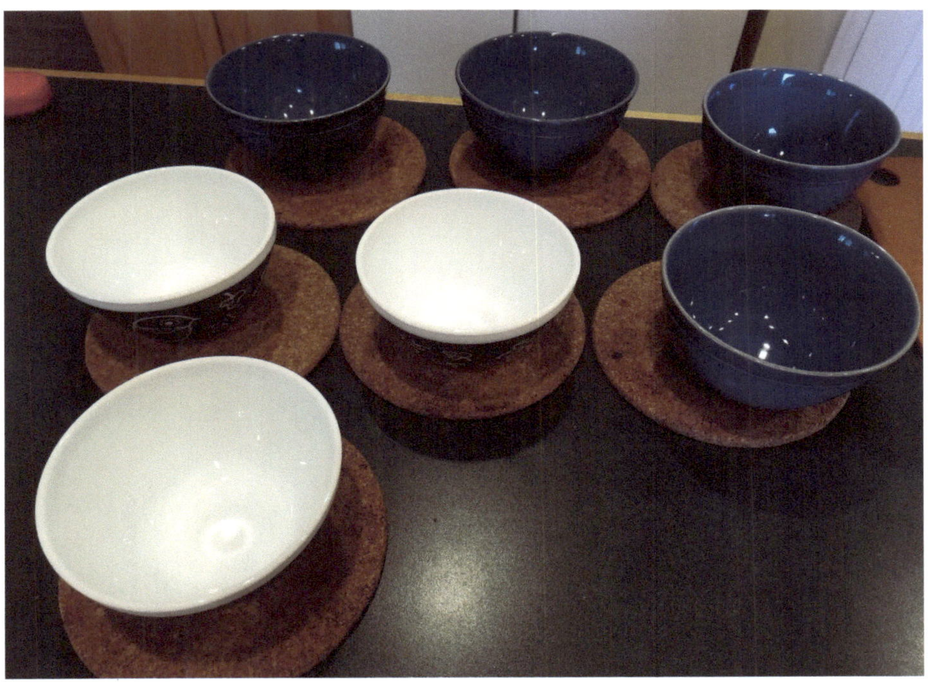

11.   Strain the broth into a large bowl.

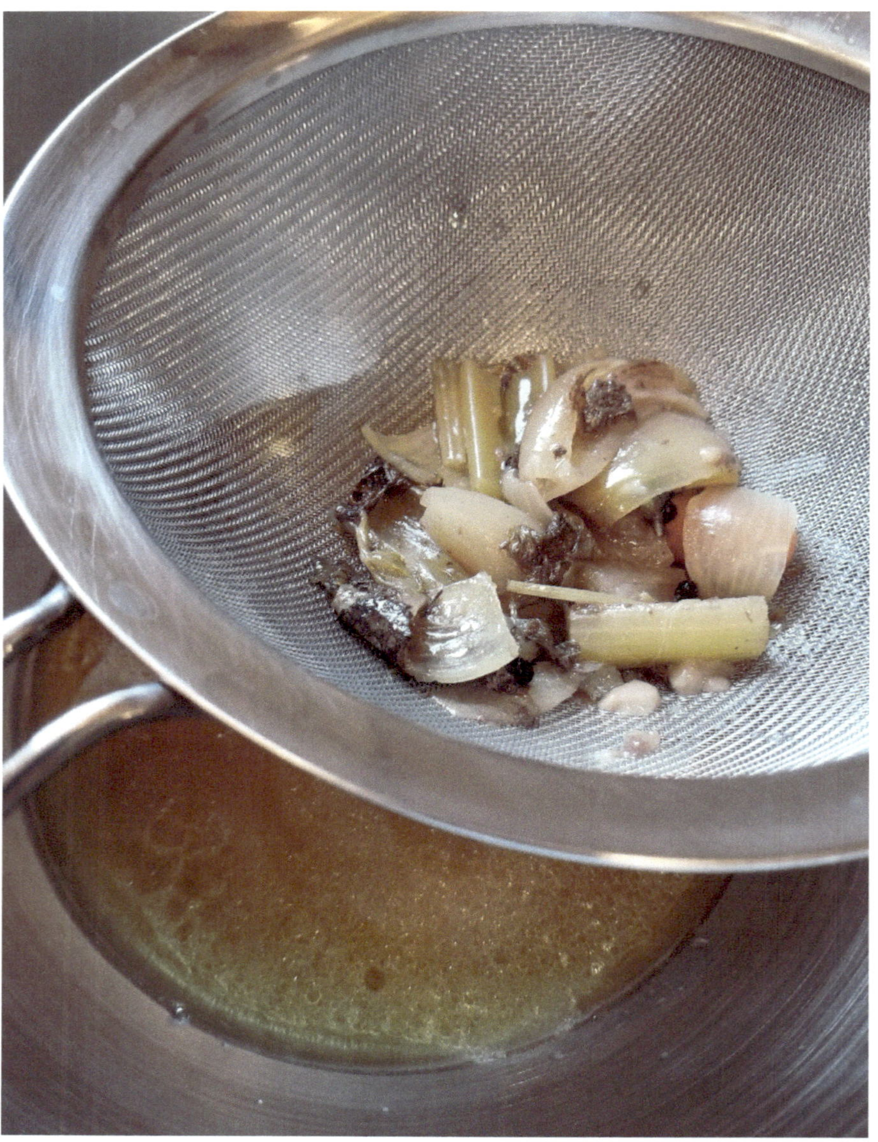

Once the broth is strained, you will notice a large amount of fat sitting on top of the broth. That looks like this:

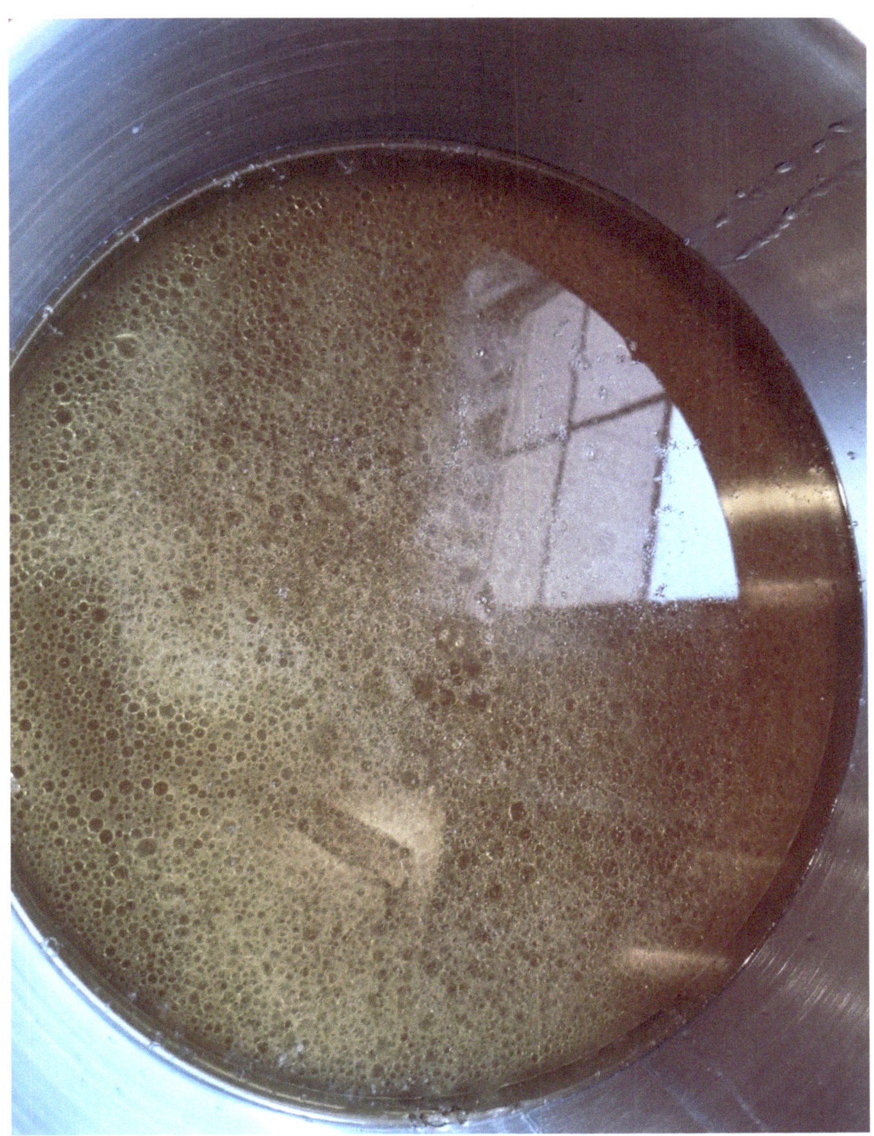

Cooling the broth looks like this:

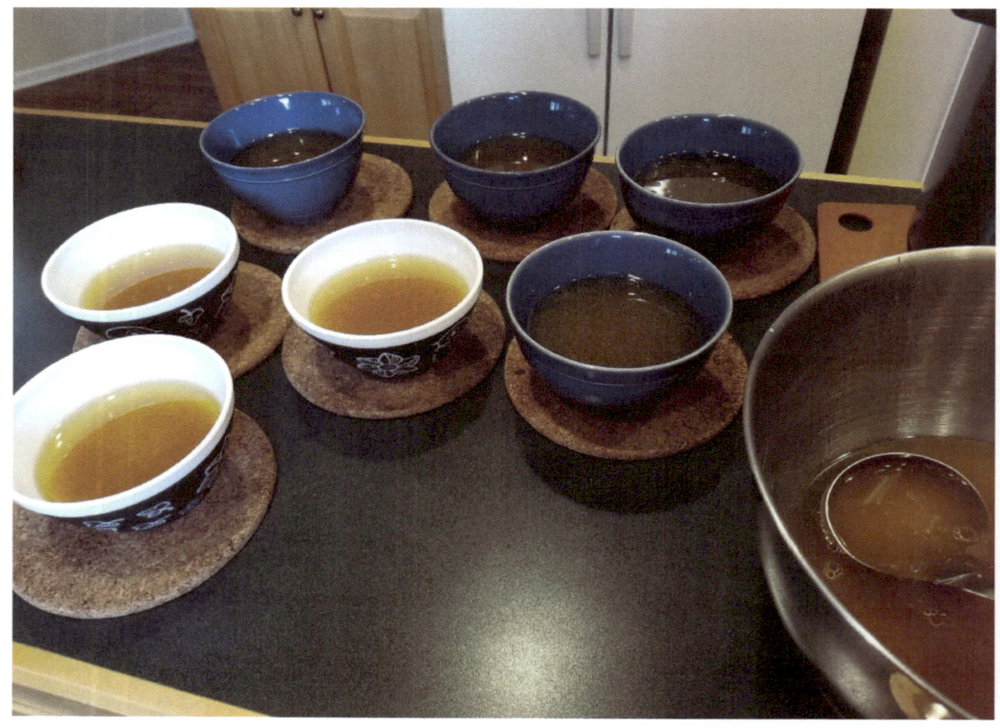

12.   Once the broth has cooled sufficiently, it is transferred to jars:

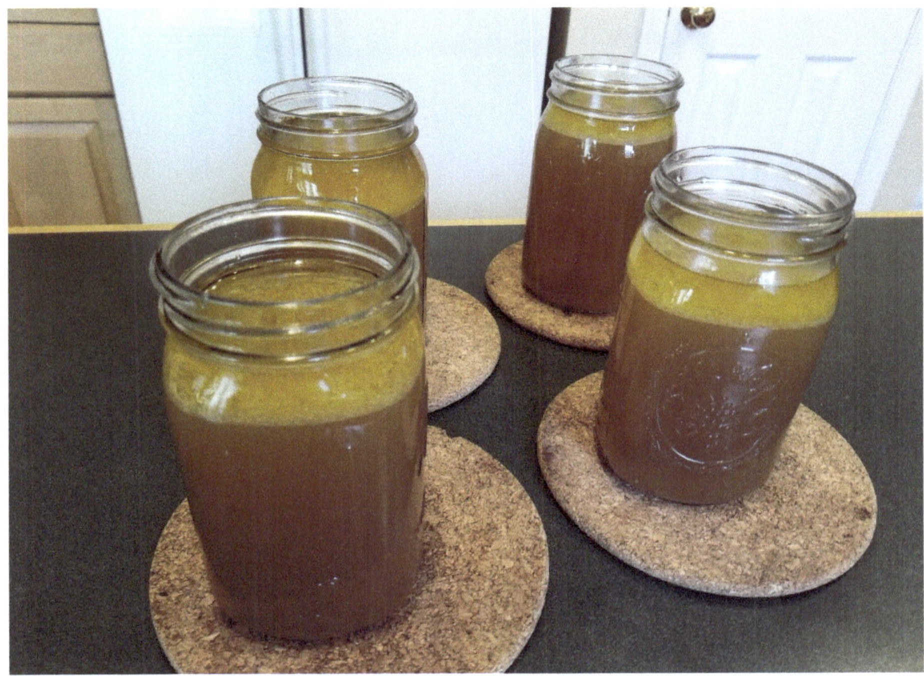

Notice the separation of the fat on top of the broth. While you won't eat this fat, it does act as a good seal. We leave it in the jars until we use the broth.

When it has cooled to room temperature, it's safe to close the jars and place them in the refrigerator.

The next morning (about 12 hours later), the jar of bone broth looks like this:

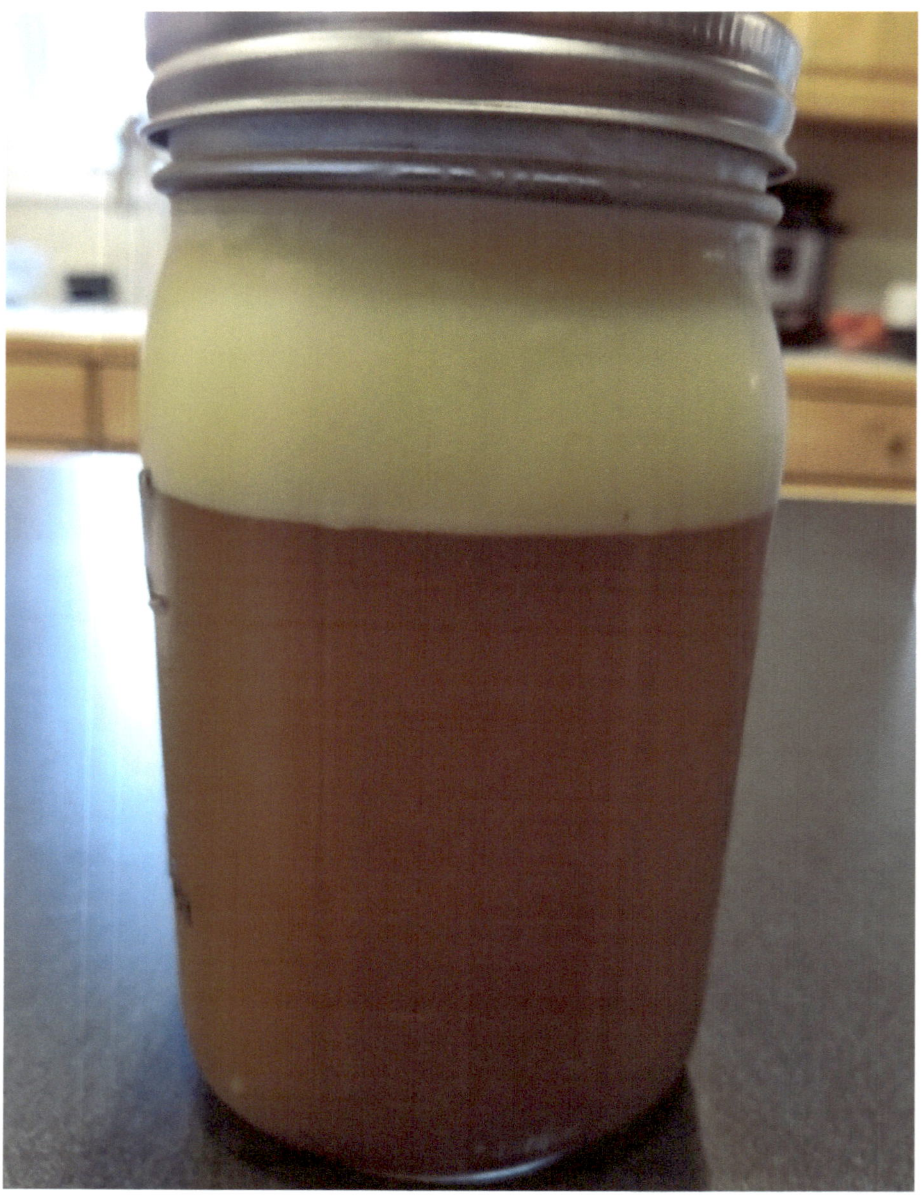

Notice how the fat has solidified, and the broth has turned to gel.

We remove the fat and store it for use later. It can be used for cooking, but we use it to make soap. The fat looks something like this:

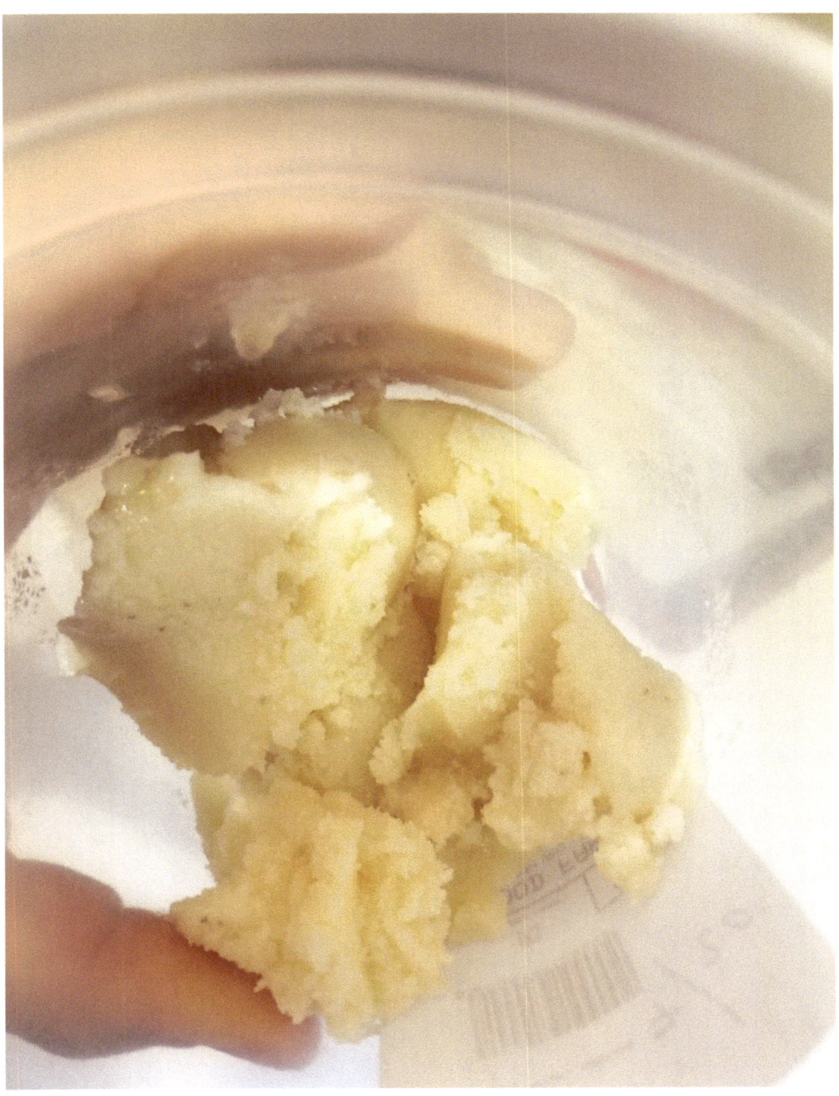

And the gel looks like this:

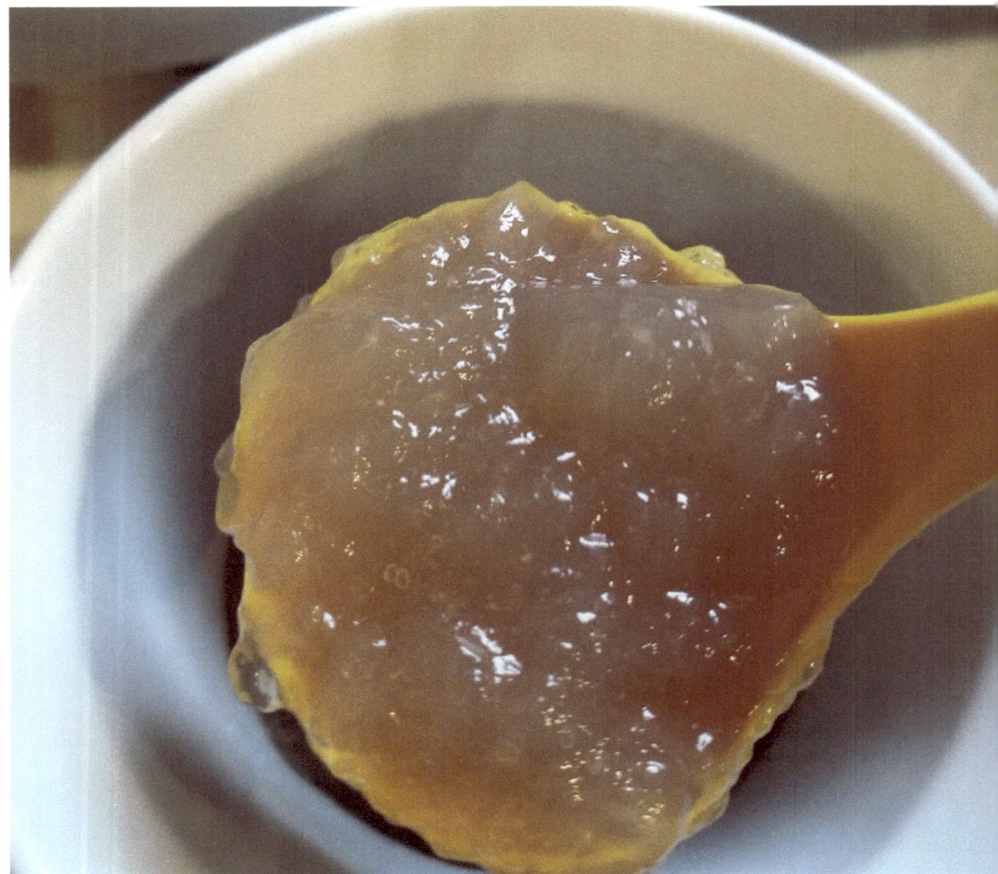

I like to sprinkle some salt and a little bit of turmeric in mine before I heat it up in the microwave.

Conclusion

I wish that I had been able to find directions like this when we started out. It took us almost six months to finally figure out how to consistently make good broth that gelled.

I wish you all the luck in the world and hope you found this guide helpful.